AMY MELISSA GUENIEVRE MCLEAN

ENERGY HEALING

Unveiling four pathways to rejuvenate our energy

This book was professionally typeset on Reedsy.
Find out more at reedsy.com

Contents

Chapter 1

ENERGY HEALING
Unveiling four ways to heal our energy

INTRODUCTION

Energy healing refers to a set of practices based on the idea that the energy flowing through the human body plays a fundamental role in physical, emotional, and spiritual health. These practices aim to rebalance this energy in order to stimulate the body's natural healing process. Whether it's Reiki, Qigong, magnetism, or Yantha, all of these methods seek to harmonize the energy flow, dissipate blockages, and restore inner balance.

The underlying principle of these practices is that every individual possesses a vital energy (called Qi, Ki, Prana, etc.) that can be disrupted by external factors such as stress, repressed emotions, or trauma. When this energy becomes imbalanced or blocked, it can lead to illness or a sense of discomfort. Energy healing, therefore, aims to restore harmony by manipulating this energy, whether through touch, meditation, physical movements, or visualizations.

Why is energy healing gaining popularity?

There are several reasons for this growing interest. First, in an increasingly stressful world, people are seeking alternatives to traditional medical treatments, looking for more holistic and natural solutions. Additionally, the growing interest in spiritual and emotional well-being, along with an increased openness to complementary therapies, has paved the way for the acceptance of these practices. Finally, an increasing number of studies suggest that certain energy healing techniques can actually improve overall well-being, further boosting their credibility and appeal.

Choosing to explore energy healing practices such as Reiki, Yantha, magnetism, and Qigong offers a unique opportunity to explore various approaches to restoring balance and vitality. Each of these methods provides a different way of working with the body's vital energy, and comparing them allows for a better understanding of their commonalities and specificities. By opening oneself to these practices, one can find the one that resonates most with personal needs, whether to relieve stress, heal emotional wounds, or improve physical health.

Reiki, a Japanese method, is based on the idea that universal energy (Ki) can be transmitted through the practitioner's hands to restore balance in the body and mind. This healing system activates the patient's natural healing potential by balancing the energy centers (chakras) and dissipating energy blockages. It is particularly appreciated for its simplicity and gentle approach.

Yantha, a lesser-known practice, is distinguished by its use of the subtle bodies and aura to assist in healing. This method combines meditation, visualization, and chakra work to rebalance inner energy. It is often used to treat emotional and spiritual issues, and its practice is deeply introspective, aiming to open the patient's consciousness to deeper levels.

Magnetism, on the other hand, uses the laying of hands to capture and redistribute the body's vital energy. Magnetizers act as conductors of energy, releasing tension and stimulating healing processes. It is highly effective for relieving physical pain or reducing stress, and is commonly used as a complement to traditional medicine.

Finally, Qigong, an ancient Chinese practice, combines physical exercises, breathing, and meditation to strengthen and circulate Qi (vital energy) within the body. Through slow, fluid movements, this practice improves energy circulation, boosts the immune system, and helps maintain a lasting state of well-being.

These four practices offer a holistic approach to healing, each with its own specifics but all aimed at restoring the body's energy balance. Their growing popularity is explained by their ability to provide natural and holistic solutions to maintain health and serenity.

Understanding Energy

Understanding Energy The Concept of Vital Energy

Vital energy, known by different names across cultures, is the fundamental essence that animates all living beings. In China, it is called Qi (or Chi), in Japan Ki, and in India Prana. This invisible but omnipresent energy flows through the universe and within our bodies, energizing our cells, organs, and tissues. It is the force that sustains life, influencing our emotions, physical health, and spiritual well-being.

The circulation of vital energy occurs through invisible channels, such as the meridians in Traditional Chinese Medicine or the chakras in Hindu traditions. This energy enters the body through energy centers (chakras) and spreads throughout the body, nourishing every organ and function. When energy flows freely and harmoniously, the body and mind are in balance, allowing one to achieve an optimal state of health.

However, blockages or imbalances in this energy flow can lead to illness, fatigue, or emotional disturbances. That is why it is essential to maintain good energy circulation, ensuring the balance of opposing forces such as Yin and Yang, or cultivating harmony between the Prana entering and leaving the body.

The importance of energy balance lies in its ability to maintain the overall health of the individual. When energy is imbalanced or stagnant, it can cause physical pain, emotional disturbances, or even chronic illness. Thus, energy healing aims to restore this balance to promote the body's natural healing process and enhance the quality of life, both physically and emotionally.

Energy Blockages and Their Impact

The flow of vital energy in our body is essential to our well-being. However, various factors can disrupt this circulation and cause energy blockages. These imbalances can result from many physical, emotional, or psychological factors. For example, prolonged stress, repressed emotions such as anger or sadness, unresolved traumas, physical injuries, or an unhealthy lifestyle can interfere with the harmony of our vital energy.

Stress is one of the main contributors to energy blockages. When a person is constantly under pressure, energy may concentrate in specific areas of the body, leading to muscle tension or chronic pain. Additionally, repressed emotions, such as fear, sadness, or anger, can create emotional blockages. These emotions, when not expressed or processed, often manifest as blockages in the chakras or meridians, affecting not only the energy balance but also the emotional and physical state of the person.

Physical injuries or traumas can also interfere with the flow of energy. After an accident or surgery, energy may become stuck in the affected area, creating stagnations that hinder healing and can cause persistent pain or movement limitations. On a more subtle level, unresolved traumatic events can create energetic scars that disrupt the flow of Qi, Ki, or Prana.

When energy does not circulate freely, it can create an imbalance that manifests in various forms of illness. For example, a blockage in the heart chakra can lead to heart or respiratory problems, while an imbalance in the solar plexus chakra may be related to digestive issues or self-confidence problems. Emotional disorders, such as anxiety, depression, or anger, are often the result of deep-seated energy imbalances.

The goal of energy healing is precisely to restore this balance by releasing blockages and promoting the free flow of energy. This can be achieved through various techniques: laying on of hands (Reiki), physical movements (Qigong), meditation, or magnetism. By rebalancing the energy, we allow the body to heal naturally and reach a state of physical, emotional, and spiritual harmony.

Reiki - Channeling Universal Energy
Origins and Principles of Reiki

Reiki has its roots in Japan at the end of the 19th century, thanks to Mikao Usui, a Buddhist monk. After studying various ancient texts and searching for a method of spiritual healing, Usui is said to have had an intense spiritual experience, which led him to discover the technique of healing through the laying on of hands. He then founded Reiki, a healing method based on the transmission of universal energy (or Ki in Japanese), a fluid and omnipresent force, to restore the balance of the body and mind.

The philosophy of Reiki is based on the idea that each individual has a connection to this universal energy. Vital energy, or Ki, flows within and around us, and healing occurs when this energy is harmonized. Reiki does not rely on supernatural powers; instead, it is a process of channeling energy through the practitioner, who acts as a conduit for transmitting this universal force to the patient.

Beyond physical healing, Reiki fosters a deep connection to oneself and to the environment. It encourages inner balance, mental peace, and compassion towards others. The practice of Reiki invites us to live in the present moment, to cultivate positive thoughts, and to strengthen the unity between body, mind, and spirit.

Today, Reiki has evolved and is practiced worldwide, not only for healing but also as a tool for personal and spiritual development.

Reiki Practices and Techniques

Reiki is practiced through several levels of initiation, each deepening the understanding and use of vital energy.

Reiki I: This is the basic level, where one learns to channel energy for oneself and others. The focus is on the laying on of hands and working with the physical body. The initiation opens the energy channels, and beginner practitioners can send energy by placing their hands on different areas of the body.

Reiki II: At this level, students learn to use specific symbols and mantras to focus and amplify the energy. These symbols (such as Cho Ku Rei to strengthen the energy or Sei He Ki for emotional balance) allow practitioners to work on a deeper level, including at a distance, for spiritual and emotional healing.

Reiki III (Master): The Master level is dedicated to teaching Reiki and transmitting energy to other practitioners. It includes advanced symbols and the initiation process to train new students.

The position of the hands in Reiki is essential. The practitioner places their hands on specific points of the body or just above it, allowing the energy to flow freely. The process of energy transmission is carried out through intention and concentration. Reiki does not involve physical force; the energy naturally directs itself to where it is needed, facilitating healing.

The Benefits of Reiki

Reiki is known for its positive effects on physical, emotional, and spiritual well-being. On the physical level, it helps reduce stress, relieve pain, and promote deep relaxation. It is used to treat conditions such as chronic pain, migraines, digestive disorders, and even to accelerate healing after surgery. By balancing energy, Reiki supports the body's natural ability to regenerate.

On the emotional level, Reiki helps release blockages related to repressed emotions such as anger, fear, or sadness. It aids in restoring emotional balance, reducing anxiety, depression, and post-traumatic stress. By bringing calm and mental clarity, it also promotes a better state of mind.

On the spiritual level, Reiki offers a deeper connection with oneself, enhancing inner serenity, intuition, and understanding of one's own spiritual nature. It helps to find inner peace, restore harmony, and cultivate mindfulness in the present moment.

Many testimonials report positive results, such as improvements in quality of life and remission of chronic conditions. However, the scientific validity of Reiki remains debated. While several studies suggest beneficial effects, such as stress reduction or improved overall well-being, there are criticisms regarding the lack of objective evidence. Reiki is often considered a complementary approach, which warrants further study in a rigorous scientific framework.

The Yantha - Balancing Energy Through the Subtle Bodies Origins and Foundations of Yantha

Yantha, a spiritual and therapeutic discipline of Tibetan origin, has its roots in the ancient traditions of the Himalayan mountains. This complex system integrates both philosophical principles and physical practices aimed at harmonizing the body, mind, and soul. Although little known in the West, it is part of the esoteric Tibetan traditions that view the human being as a network of interconnected energies, constantly interacting with the universe.

At the heart of Yantha lies a deep understanding of the subtle bodies—these energetic layers that, beyond the physical body, govern our well-being and our interactions with the world. These subtle bodies include the astral body, the mental body, and the spiritual body, each influencing the individual's overall health. The aura, the luminous emanation surrounding every being, is seen as a reflection of the inner balance or imbalance. A clear and radiant aura symbolizes a person in harmony with themselves, while a dull or fragmented aura may indicate emotional or spiritual disturbances.

Yantha, in its modern form, adapts to contemporary needs by offering healing methods based on the re-harmonization of these subtle energies. These practices aim to restore balance to the aura and strengthen the subtle bodies, allowing the individual to regain health, serenity, and mental clarity.

The Healing Techniques of Yantha

Yantha is based on a set of healing techniques that directly affect the subtle energies of the body. Among the most fundamental practices are work on the chakras and energy meridians. The chakras, energy centers located along the spine, are considered points of convergence between the physical body and the subtle bodies. Each chakra regulates a specific aspect of the being, such as emotions, thought, or vitality. Yantha aims to rebalance these energy centers by releasing blockages that can lead to disease or emotional imbalances.

Energy meridians, invisible channels in the body, carry the vital energy, known as "chi." When a meridian is blocked, it can cause energy stagnation, affecting physical and emotional health. Working on these meridians, through techniques such as pressure, massage, or energetic manipulation, helps restore the harmonious flow of energy.

Meditation, visualization, and intention also play a crucial role in the Yantha healing process. Meditation helps calm the mind and connect more deeply with subtle energies. Visualization involves imagining healing energy flows circulating through the chakras and meridians, thus facilitating rebalancing. Finally, conscious and directed intention is a powerful tool: it channels the energy and directs the healing process, amplifying the effects of the other techniques. Combined, these practices restore a deep harmony between the body and mind.

The Benefits and Applications of Yantha

Yantha offers a holistic approach to healing, addressing the root causes of spiritual, mental, and emotional imbalances. By balancing the subtle bodies, this practice promotes spiritual healing by allowing the individual to reconnect with their deep essence and spiritual dimension. This re-harmonization creates a sense of inner peace and clarity, which is essential for personal growth.

From a mental and emotional perspective, Yantha helps release the energetic blockages that underpin negative feelings such as anxiety, depression, or stress. Through meditation and visualization practices, this approach strengthens emotional stability, improves concentration, and helps regain a positive attitude toward life.

Yantha also stands out for its ability to prevent and treat chronic illnesses. By regulating the energy flow and rebalancing the meridians and chakras, it helps prevent the onset of diseases while supporting the healing process of existing conditions. Unlike other energy therapies that may focus solely on specific symptoms, Yantha takes a comprehensive approach, aiming to restore balance to the body and mind as a whole.

Finally, Yantha distinguishes itself from other forms of energy healing through its deep connection to Tibetan traditions and its unique combination of physical, meditative, and intentional practices, making it a particularly complete and powerful approach.

Magnetism - The Art of Transferring Energy through the Laying on of Hands Origins and Foundations of Magnetism

Magnetism, in its therapeutic form, has its roots in the 18th century with Franz Anton Mesmer, an Austrian physician, who introduced the concept of the "magnetic fluid." Mesmer believed that this universal fluid circulated throughout the body and could be manipulated to restore energetic balance and heal certain ailments. Although his theories were controversial and often seen as mystical, he paved the way for the exploration of subtle energy and its impact on human health.

In the 19th century, magnetism evolved into hypnosis and magnetic somnambulism thanks to pioneers such as James Braid and Jean-Martin Charcot, who developed more rigorous methods to study and apply magnetism. However, it was in the 20th century that the practice of magnetism modernized, with a deeper understanding of vital energy and energy fields.

Today, magnetism is often approached through the lens of vital energy and human energetics, where every living being is surrounded by interconnected energy fields. Modern practice is based on the idea that the human body emits an electromagnetic field and that this field can be influenced by other fields, whether biological or external. Magnetism techniques aim to rebalance this energy field, thereby facilitating self-healing and promoting physical and mental well-being.

Contemporary science is beginning to explore quantum physics and electromagnetic waves to explain the phenomena observed in energy practices, thus bringing magnetism closer to modern scientific discoveries.

The Practice of Magnetism

The practice of magnetism is based on the use of subtle energies to restore the body's energetic balance. One of the most common techniques is the laying on of hands, where the magnetizer places their hands near the patient's body or on specific areas to capture and transmit energy. This method is based on the idea that the magnetizer can perceive energetic imbalances and redirect vital energy in order to restore harmony.

Another technique used is energy sweeping, which involves passing the hands over the patient's body, often in a fluid motion, without direct contact. The magnetizer "sweeps" away stagnant or disturbed energies, removing them to allow for better circulation of vital energy. This process helps to release energetic blockages and promotes healing.

The magnetizer captures the surrounding energy, often by entering a state of concentration and receptivity. Depending on the practice, they may use their hands as receptors to "capture" energy from the universe or the environment. They then redirect this energy to the patient through their hands or by their intention, acting as a channel between the source of energy and the person receiving the treatment. The fluidity of this transfer depends on the magnetizer's ability to stay connected to their own energy field and maintain a clear intention for healing.

These techniques aim to rebalance the energy flows, thereby promoting physical, mental, and emotional healing.

The Benefits of Magnetism

Magnetism, as an energetic practice, is renowned for its therapeutic benefits on both the body and the mind. One of the most frequently reported effects is pain relief. By rebalancing the energies, this method can reduce chronic pain, such as that associated with arthritis or muscle injuries. Magnetism helps to release both physical and emotional tensions, contributing to an overall sense of well-being.

It is also effective for stress management. By calming the nervous system, magnetism promotes a state of deep relaxation, thereby reducing symptoms related to anxiety and daily stress. This process helps restore emotional balance and inner serenity.

Another notable application of magnetism is the improvement of energy circulation. By unblocking the meridians and harmonizing the chakras, it allows for better flow of vital energy throughout the body, which can strengthen the immune system and improve overall health.

Many testimonials report positive results, including pain reduction and improved mood. However, despite these positive experiences, the lack of direct scientific evidence limits the universal recognition of magnetism in traditional medicine. The benefits are often perceived subjectively, depending on the individual, and may vary from person to person, which contributes to a shared perception of this practice.

The Qigong - Cultivating and Circulating Energy Through the Body Origins and Principles of Qigong

Qigong, an ancient practice, has its roots in ancient China, where it evolved alongside traditional Chinese medicine (TCM). The term "Qigong" is composed of two words: Qi (vital energy) and Gong (work or mastery), which literally means "work of energy." Qigong has been practiced for health, longevity, and inner harmony, playing a key role in the prevention and treatment of various illnesses. It is closely linked to traditional Chinese medicine, which is based on the circulation of energy through the body's meridians. When balanced, Qi allows the body to function optimally, while its blockage or imbalance can lead to health issues.

In the context of Qigong, Qi represents the vital energy present in every individual and in the universe. This energy circulates through the body via channels called meridians, and Qigong seeks to promote its harmonious movement. The fundamental principle of Qigong lies in the alignment of the body, mind, and energy. Through gentle physical exercises, controlled breathing, and mental concentration, the practitioner cultivates harmony between these three aspects.

This not only strengthens the internal energy but also maintains a state of overall health and well-being, fostering balance and serenity.

27

The Practices of Qigong

Qigong is divided into several forms, each with a specific goal. The three main types are therapeutic Qigong, martial Qigong, and spiritual Qigong.

Therapeutic Qigong: This form is used to maintain or restore health. It includes gentle exercises designed to balance the flow of Qi (vital energy) in the body. These practices are often tailored to individual needs and can address specific conditions by regulating the internal organs and harmonizing the meridians.

Martial Qigong: Used in Chinese martial arts, martial Qigong develops internal strength, endurance, and power. It includes more dynamic movements and specific postures that strengthen the body and mind, enabling an increase in available energy for martial practice.

Spiritual Qigong: This form focuses on cultivating the mind and consciousness. It aims to harmonize the body, mind, and energy to achieve a state of deep serenity, meditation, and spiritual development.

Breathing techniques are at the core of all forms of Qigong. Abdominal (or diaphragmatic) breathing helps calm the mind and increase energy.

Slow, fluid body movements promote the circulation of Qi, while meditation aids in concentration, introspection, and energetic alignment. These combined practices offer benefits for the body, mind, and soul.

The Benefits of Qigong

Qigong is renowned for its numerous benefits on both physical and mental health. By strengthening the immune system, it helps prevent illness by stimulating the circulation of Qi and regulating energy throughout the body. Regular practice also improves stress management by activating the parasympathetic nervous system, promoting relaxation, and reducing symptoms of anxiety and tension. Vitality is further enhanced through the harmonization of the body, mind, and energy, allowing for a sustained level of energy throughout the day.

Many testimonies report the effectiveness of Qigong in treating chronic conditions such as arthritis, diabetes, and fibromyalgia. Practitioners often experience a significant reduction in pain, improved mobility, and an overall improvement in well-being. Studies also show that Qigong can have positive effects in managing cardiovascular and respiratory disorders by increasing oxygenation and strengthening respiratory muscles.

Qigong is increasingly finding its place in modern medicine, complementing conventional treatments. In the West, the practice of Qigong is gaining growing recognition, with a marked interest in alternative medicine. Attitudes are gradually shifting, and Qigong is now seen as an effective way to prevent disease and enhance quality of life, beyond just healing.

Common Points Between the Practices

Energy practices such as Qigong, magnetism, Yantha, and Reiki share common principles, notably the activation of universal energy and the balance of energy flows throughout the body. Each method is based on the idea that vital energy, although often invisible, flows within and around us, influencing our physical, mental, and spiritual health.

In Qigong, vital energy, or Qi, is cultivated through slow movements, breathing exercises, and meditative practices. Reiki, on the other hand, focuses on the laying on of hands to channel universal energy and direct it where it is needed. Magnetism and Yantha function similarly, using the hands or intention to capture and redirect energy. The goal is always to restore the body's energetic balance.

Conscious intention and meditation play a central role in all of these practices. Through meditation, the mind is calmed, allowing energy to flow more freely and harmoniously. Intention becomes a powerful tool to guide this energy and promote healing. Furthermore, the balance of chakras (in Reiki and Yantha) or meridians (in Qigong and magnetism) is crucial for optimal health, with each system aiming to harmonize and release energy blockages, whether physical or emotional.

Fundamental Differences

Although Qigong, Reiki, magnetism, and Yantha share a common goal—energetic balance and healing—their cultural approaches, techniques, and underlying philosophies vary considerably.

Qigong, originating from China, is rooted in traditional Chinese medicine and is based on the idea that vital energy, or Qi, flows through the body along meridians. Its practices combine physical movements, breathing exercises, and meditation to harmonize the energy flow, prevent illness, and promote healing.

Reiki, a Japanese practice, focuses on the laying on of hands to channel universal energy. Practitioners use intention to direct this energy to areas of the body that need healing. Unlike Qigong, Reiki does not require physical movements but instead focuses on relaxation and energetic rebalancing through intention.

Magnetism, often considered a Western approach, also uses the laying on of hands, but lacks the formal structure found in Reiki or Qigong. It is based on the idea that energy can be transferred between the practitioner and the patient to restore energetic balance.

Yantha, while similar to Reiki in its manipulation of energy, relies on a unique spiritual philosophy influenced by Tibetan traditions, and seeks to align the patient's subtle bodies.

Thus, while these practices aim to balance energy and promote healing, their techniques and philosophies differ depending on the cultures and belief systems behind them.

Choosing the Practice that Suits You

Choosing an energy healing method depends on several personal factors, such as your specific needs, spiritual beliefs, and individual preferences. Each energy practice—whether Qigong, Reiki, magnetism, or Yantha—offers distinct approaches to promoting healing.

If you are looking to balance your vital energy and improve your physical vitality, Qigong could be a good option. This Chinese practice, which combines body movements, breathing, and meditation, is ideal for strengthening the immune system and promoting overall bodily harmony. Reiki, on the other hand, may be suitable if you are seeking emotional or spiritual healing. It relies on the laying on of hands and the intention to channel universal energy, offering a gentle and relaxing approach.

Magnetism is often chosen for its immediate effects on pain management or stress relief. If you prefer a less structured method with a strong component of energy transfer, it may be a good choice. Finally, if you are drawn to a deeper spiritual approach related to the subtle bodies and the harmonization of energies, Yantha might appeal to you, especially if you are sensitive to Tibetan traditions.

Taking your personal beliefs and feelings into account is essential. If a practice speaks to you intuitively, it is likely the one that will suit you best. It may be helpful to try different methods and observe which one resonates with you the most.

The Future of Energy Healing

The future of energy healing looks promising, with a growing recognition of its effectiveness and a gradual integration into both traditional and complementary healthcare. Practices such as Reiki, Qigong, magnetism, and Yantha, long considered alternatives, are gaining credibility thanks to an increasing number of scientific studies exploring their impact on stress management, pain reduction, and emotional balance.

More and more, these practices are being integrated into hospitals, clinics, and wellness centers as complementary treatments to conventional medical care. Reiki, for example, is now used in some hospitals to help patients relax, manage pain, and strengthen their immune system, especially in the context of cancer treatment. Qigong and magnetism are also finding their place in rehabilitation programs and in the prevention of chronic diseases.

One of the key challenges for the future of energy healing will be to combine ancient knowledge with modern scientific advancements. Additional clinical studies on the effectiveness of these practices could pave the way for integrative medicine, where energy-based and conventional approaches complement each other to promote holistic health. Education and awareness for both the general public and healthcare professionals will be essential for broader adoption and a better understanding of these beneficial practices.

Conclusion

Energy is the vital force that flows through us and connects us to everything around us. By understanding and harmonizing it, we can create deep balance in both our bodies and minds. Energy practices such as Reiki, Qigong, magnetism, and Yantha remind us of the importance of working with this energy to maintain good health and lasting well-being. By taking care of our vital energy, we can not only prevent illness but also improve our vitality, manage stress, and support faster and more complete healing.

In our daily lives, we are constantly exposed to energetic influences — stress, emotions, and our environment. If these influences are not properly managed, they can disrupt our energy flow and lead to imbalances. This is why it becomes essential to realign our energy regularly, by adopting energy healing practices that help restore this natural balance. These methods are not only solutions for physical ailments, but also powerful tools for emotional and mental well-being.

I invite you to explore these energy practices and experience their potential. Perhaps you will feel the positive effects on your body, mind, and life. Trust your intuition and your needs. Each practice has its own specifics, but all aim to restore harmony and reconnect you to your original energy. It is not just about healing, but about living mindfully and embracing your inner power. Experiment, explore, and discover the benefits of energy healing that resonates with you.

Hope you will explore those practices, and give me feedback on your experiment with your review on amazon, take care.

Resources

Books and specialized works

"The Art of Reiki: Teachings of Mikao Usui" by Mikao Usui and William Lee Rand

This book is a combination of the traditional teachings of Mikao Usui and modern perspectives on Reiki.

"Reiki Energy Medicine: Bringing Healing Touch into Home, Hospital, and Hospice" by Frans Stiene

This book explores the scientific foundations of Reiki and discusses its use in medical settings, as well as current research on its therapeutic effects.

"Yantha: The Tibetan Healing Art" by Tenzin Wangyal Rinpoche

This book explains the practice of Yantha and its connection to Tibetan spiritual traditions, particularly the alignment of the subtle bodies and the use of energy for healing. It also places these practices in perspective with cultural and philosophical differences from other energy healing modalities.

"The Energetic Body: How to Use Your Subtle Bodies for Healing" by James W. Van Praagh

While this book focuses on subtle bodies in general rather than specifically on Yantha, it provides a detailed insight into the aura, chakras, and energetic bodies, which can be helpful in better understanding the concept of energetic balance in Yantha.

"Mesmerism and the American Cure of Souls" by Philip M. Davis

This book explores the history of mesmerism, particularly the work of Mesmer and his influence on medicine and psychology.

"The Healing Power of Energy Medicine" by Donna Eden and David Feinstein

A modern work that details vital energy, human energy fields, and how energy practices, such as magnetism, influence health.

"The Physics of Healing" by Gary E. Schwartz and Linda G. S.

This book examines the scientific foundations behind energy healing practices, including magnetism.

"Qigong for Health and Vitality" by Rodney A. Carter

A book on Qigong that explains the underlying principles of this practice and how it helps rebalance the body's energy to improve overall health.

"Energy Medicine: The Science and Mystery of Healing" by Donna Eden

This book explains how energy influences health and healing, offering practical advice on working with the body's energy through techniques such as magnetism and other energy approaches.

"The Root of Chinese Qigong: Secrets of Health, Longevity, & Enlightenment" by Jingyu Li

This book provides a detailed introduction to the history of Qigong, particularly its connections with traditional Chinese medicine, and offers an in-depth explanation of the fundamental principles of Qi and vital energy in this practice.

Scientific articles and research

"Effects of Reiki on Pain and Anxiety in the Cancer Patient: A Systematic Review of the Literature" (Journal of Alternative and Complementary Medicine)

This article reviews scientific studies on the effects of Reiki on symptoms such as pain, stress, and anxiety in cancer patients.

"Mesmerism and the Development of Hypnosis" by Ernest Hilgard

This article analyzes Mesmer's theories and their evolution into modern hypnosis, outlining the scientific history behind mesmerism.

"Biofields: A Conceptual Model" by William Tiller, John P. Schauble, et al. (Journal of Scientific Exploration, 1995)

This article discusses biological energy fields and how they may interact with the environment and other fields.

"Healing with the Hands: A Study of Energy Transfer" by Catherine L. Hall et al. This article explores the mechanisms of hands-on healing, detailing how energy is perceived and transferred during magnetism sessions.

"The Role of Qi in Qigong: A Theoretical Approach" by David W. K. Ho (Journal of Chinese Medicine)

This academic article explains in detail the role of Qi in Qigong and how its flow through the body can affect health and well-being. It also provides theoretical explanations on the alignment of energy, body, and mind.

"The Role of Qigong in Traditional Chinese Medicine: A Therapeutic Approach" by Y. Z. Liu et al. (Journal of Traditional Chinese Medicine)

This article explores the various applications of Qigong within the framework of Traditional Chinese Medicine, including its therapeutic role and the different forms practiced in a medical context.

"Qigong and Health: Benefits and Applications" in *The Journal of Alternative and Complementary Medicine*

This study examines the impact of therapeutic Qigong on health, breathing techniques, movements, and their role in enhancing physical and mental well-being.

"Comparative Analysis of Qigong, Reiki, and Magnetic Healing" (Journal of Complementary and Alternative Medicine) This article presents a comparative analysis of energy healing practices, studying the differences in techniques.

Specialized websites

Reiki.org – reiki.org

This website is a comprehensive resource on Reiki, featuring information on its history, practices, benefits, and testimonials from practitioners. It also offers courses and certifications for levels ranging from beginner to master.

Tenzin Wangyal Rinpoche's Website – ligmincha.org

Tenzin Wangyal Rinpoche, an expert in Yantha, offers numerous resources on this Tibetan practice, including explanations of its spiritual foundations and its differences from other forms of energy healing.

The Energy Body: Exploring the Subtle Body - Articles on Mind Body Green

An introductory article that explores the energetic concepts of the aura, chakras, and subtle bodies, which are essential for understanding Yantha and similar energy healing practices.

Institute of Noetic Sciences (IONS) – noetic.org

IONS explores the science of consciousness and energy phenomena, including magnetism and its therapeutic applications.

The Chinese Medicine & Qigong Center – qihealing.com

This website offers educational articles on Qi and Qigong, including explanations on the energetic alignment of the body and the principles of Traditional Chinese Medicine.

Energy Medicine Institute – energymedicineinstitute.com

This site offers training, articles, and resources on various energy healing practices, including magnetism and the body's energetic systems.

Online testimonials

"Personal Stories of Reiki Healing" on healingexperiences.org This website features testimonials from individuals who have experienced Reiki and other energy healing practices to treat chronic conditions and improve their quality of life.

"Personal Stories of Healing through Magnetism" on healingexpe

riences.org

This website features testimonials from individuals who have experienced magnetism sessions, highlighting the positive effects on pain, stress, and overall well-being, while also mentioning variations in outcomes.

"Personal Stories of Qigong Healing" on healingexperiences.org

This website presents testimonials from individuals who have used Qigong to manage chronic conditions such as cancer, nervous system disorders, and chronic pain.